LOSE WEIGHT NOW BY FASTING

An Essential Guide To Intermittent Fasting

By
Star Blessings

Table of Contents

Book Description 1

Introduction 2

    Obesity Epidemic 3

What is Intermittent Fasting? 6

    Intermittent fasting as a lifestyle 7

    Cheat Day 7

    The Scale 9

Ideal Intermittent Fasting Plan 10

    Alternate day fasting (ADF) 10

    Meal-skipping 12

    Eat Stop Eat 13

    Lean gains (16/8 method) 15

    Warrior Diet 18

    5:2 diet 20

Weight Loss Through Intermittent Fasting 21

Benefits of Intermittent Fasting 24

    Lowers Risk of Type 2 Diabetes 24

    Reduces Oxidative Stress and Inflammation 24

    Lower Risk of Heart Disease 25

    Cellular Repair 25

    Prevent Cancer 25

    Brain Health 25

    Prevent Alzheimer's Disease 26

Extend Lifespan 26

Tips for Beginners..28

    Try Fasting After Dinner 28

    Difference between Boredom and Hunger 29

    Drink Water 29

    Skip Flavored Drinks..30

    Consume Protein...31

    Avoid Unhealthy Foods..31

    Take it Slow 32

Who Shouldn't Try Intermittent Fasting?..33

    People Suffering from an Eating Disorder 33

    Pregnant Women 33

    People suffering from Type 1 Diabetes 34

    Athletes in Training 34

Side Effects of Intermittent Fasting 35

Frequently Asked Questions 37

    Can I Drink Liquids While Fasting?...37

    Is it Unhealthy to Skip Breakfast?..37

    Can I Take Supplements While Fasting? 37

    Can I Exercise While Fasting? 37

    Will I Lose My Muscles If I Fast?...38

    Will Fasting Slow Down My Metabolism..38

    Will I suffer from starvation mode? 38

    Can my child try intermittent fasting?..38

Conclusion 39

Book Description

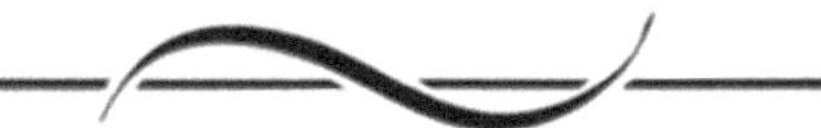

The way you choose to live your daily life is a part of who you are. The things you practice defines your values and skills. In the same way, the diet you choose to have defines what you want to seek out in your life.

Intermittent fasting is a word that you must have heard before. It is not something new and has been practiced for decades, either due to physical health reasons, religious or even mental health reasons.

Control of your schedule means having control of your life. Thus, this book has been created for you so that you can do all of this in the best way possible. Continue to read, and you will be introduced to a lifestyle that you could have never imagined existed.

Introduction

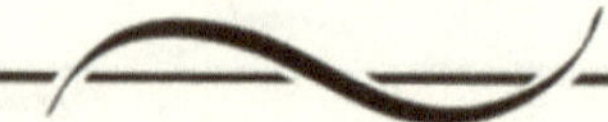

Intermittent fasting is not something you hear in your everyday conversations, but it is something you would be recommended if you decided to take on a healthy diet.

If you have never heard of this phrase before, then it would be quite surprising as intermittent fasting is now the world's most popular diet plan and fitness trend.

People all around the world have started looking into this diet to improve their health (both physically and mentally) as well as make their lifestyle a little easier.

Many studies have shown the positive effects of intermittent fasting on an individual's body and brain. It is said to even prolong one's lifespan if done properly.

In simple words, intermittent fasting is a cycle of eating patterns that has stages where you fast (meaning you stop eating) and where you eat. There is no specific food chart that you must follow, as this diet involves only the timing you should be eating at and not what you should be eating.

So, if you really think about it, intermittent fasting is not even a diet; it is more of an eating pattern. This eating pattern is not something you should take lightly because although it is not a diet, it is still a lifestyle that needs to be followed strictly for you to see any sort of result.

However, don't get intimidated as once you make up your mind about this new lifestyle; you will slowly learn to form a proper plan for yourself in no time.

Do not think that your body will continuously be in starvation mode as fasting has been a part of our daily practice since humans existed. There were no supermarkets, refrigerators, or an abundance of food before. In the past, humans could fast for a period of time before they could finally find food for the day, so intermittent fasting is not something new; it just hasn't been explored by you.

Fasting from time to time is more natural than eating 24 hours a day. It is better not to always eat 3-4 meals, especially if your physical activities are less. But like it was said before, intermittent fasting has nothing to do with what you consume.

Obesity Epidemic

Obesity is no longer something we can take lightly. It has risen so fast over the last few decades that it is now an international crisis. If you were to define obesity or overweight, then you could say it is the accumulation of excess fast within an individual's body to an abnormal level and can lead to one's death.

In order to claim that someone is obese, one must observe their Body Mass Index (BMI). BMI is a simple index that uses an individual's weight-for-height and is often used to classify someone as overweight or obese. To calculate a person's BMI, one should take their weight in kilograms and divide it by the square of their height, which should be in meters (Kg/M^2).

The cause behind obesity is simple, it is due to not having a balanced amount of calories consumed and calories used. All around the world, the intake of food that has a lot of energy has increased. Such foods are also high in fat and sugars.

The World Health Organization (WHO) defines adults as overweight once they have hit a BMI of more than or equal to 25. While a BMI of more than or equal to 30 is considered as obesity.

However, do not take BMI as your only indication for obesity as it is just a rough guide to calculate the general health of a population in total since the same BMI applies to both genders who are considered to be adults.

Sometimes your BMI is high due to increased muscle mass. An increase in muscle mass does not mean you have become obese since obesity is correlated to fats, not muscles.

Even in childhood, obesity has shown a considerable amount of growth in the past few decades.

In 2019, 38.2 million children (estimated value) who were under the age of five had been either overweight or had been diagnosed with obesity.

This issue was considered to be a part of high-income countries, but now even low to middle-income countries are suffering from obesity, especially those individuals that live in urban settings.

There are several problems that an individual can be facing due to obesity, such as:

- Cardiovascular diseases (heart disease/stroke): this was the leading cause of death in 2012.
- Musculoskeletal disorders
- Several types of cancer examples include endometrial, breast, ovarian, prostate, liver, gallbladder, and kidney)

All of these diseases are considered non-communicable diseases, and their risk increase as the BMI of a person increases.

Having a supportive environment to guide you through life is extremely important. Communities help people make choices and shape them as individuals. By making good food and diet choice, one can truly change their life in an instant.

This is why intermittent fasting can be used to build a community so that you do not feel alone in your goal to achieve a certain lifestyle as many people might plan some events that you cannot participate in since you are fasting.

Becoming overweight or obese is a choice, and so is taking the right step to set a proper lifestyle. In some cases, gaining weight is due to medical reasons, but the majority of people become obese or overweight due to their own life choices.

To build a community that helps everyone, you along with the people you care for can:

- reduce intake of fat and sugar
- Increase consumption of vegetables and fruits

- Engage in physical activities

No doubt there are so many other factors that are encouraging this growth in obesity rates, such as the food industry that promotes unhealthy eating habit, but they too can play a role in reducing obesity by:

- Reducing high sugar, salt, and fat in their processed foods
- Including proper nutrition's in their foods
- Making healthy foods more affordable for people
- Adding a high tax on sugary drinks

People won't ever change for you, but you can change for yourself. So if you wish to take a stand for your own life, then the right time is now.

What is Intermittent Fasting?

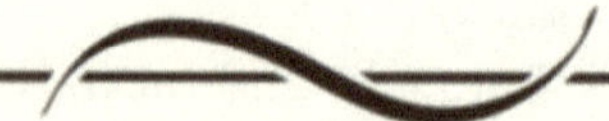

Fasting is different than starvation. In what way? You may be thinking well; it differs in one crucial way: control. Starvation is an involuntary absence of food; sometimes, it may even be voluntary. You could say starvation is neither deliberate neither is it controlled, and it can lead to death.

On the other hand, intermittent fasting is an action you do by choice since it is an avoidance of food due to health, religious or spiritual reasons.

If you do it right, you will not suffer from exhaustion, pain, and certainly not death.

In intermittent fasting, food is available for you. However, in this case, you choose not to eat it as you practice self-control. The fast can be for as long as you want it to be, such as not eating for eight hours, sixteen hours, or a whole day.

You can start your fast any time or day of the week, and you can also end the fast at your own will.

You can also go on without eating for a whole week, but no one would recommend this strategy as it can cause weakness over time.

At any time where you are not consuming food, you are indirectly fasting. Let's take one example; you are fasting from dinner to breakfast the next day as there is a huge time gap in between, approximately eight hours, where you are not consuming any food.

So if you look at it this way, then intermittent fasting is going to be considered as a part of your life either directly or indirectly.

You could say intermittent fasting is one of the oldest and most well-known dietary interventions imaginable. Take the term "Breakfast" this literally means breaking your fast, and you do this daily.

Even the English language implies that you should have a period of fasting, and it should be done every day, even if it is only for a few hours. This isn't something painful, nor is it a punishment; it is just a good habit to build.

Somehow we have overlooked the capabilities of intermittent fasting. It has so much power to change an individual's life and several other therapeutic potentials.

Remember, this is an option for us to choose, not for someone else to choose for us.

Intermittent fasting as a lifestyle

Consumption of food is done every day, and for us, this "activity" is fairly simple but extremely hard to balance. We tend to overeat several times throughout the day, and this has a huge effect on our health.

The main obstacle we face in terms of eating healthy is the work that we must put into our daily meals.

Eating healthy is not the hard part; it's making healthy food for ourselves every day that puts people off when it comes to taking care of their health.

However, if you take on intermittent fasting, life will become so much easier as you do not have to plan, cook, prep, or clean up as much as you would usually do since you do not spend half the day eating food.

This is why intermittent fasting is considered to be a life hack, as it not only simplifies things in terms of food and health, but it also gives you the feeling of getting your life together.

Cheat Day

Cheat day is a word you will have to remove from your dictionary. You are not in a relationship with intermittent fasting, so you can't say you are going to cheat. You keep cheat days when you are dieting. But you don't diet during intermittent fasting because it is not a diet, it is a lifestyle.

Its simple cheating is a negative word in your life now. We shouldn't be cheating in the first place, so why keep a "cheat day" in your lifestyle?

Many people ask this question: "Can I have a cheat day when I am fasting?" the answer is no, you can't have a cheat day. Cheating is related to guilt, and intermittent fasting is not made for you to feel guilty. Intermittent fasting does not even have a diet plan.

The only thing involved in intermittent fasting is timing. These "timings" are when you are consuming your daily food intake. So intermittent fasting just involves a small period of food consumption and then a period of fasting.

Cheat days are kept by those who can't consume the things they want to on a daily basis. This is because they go through a period of guilt once they have consumed the thing they were craving.

Thus, in order to avoid this guilt, an individual will keep one day where they allow themselves to eat whatever they want.

But you do not need to have to be feeling guilty about anything. That mindset can be exhausting, and because of that, it is hard to maintain that sort of a lifestyle where anything you consume makes you doubt whether or not it was the right choice.

In intermittent fasting, you control everything; if you wish to keep a close eye on what you eat during your eating time, then go ahead, do it. But it is not something you will absolutely have to do since you are in control.

Cheat days usually end on a bad note. Your body is always giving you signals at the end of the day that it does not feel good at all, and this leads you to feel uncomfortable throughout the night. Once you go from a clean diet to one where you consume all the fatty and sugary foods all at once, it can take a huge toll on the body.

On special occasions, it is okay for you to divert your attention away from intermittent fasting. It is your choice to pick whatever time suits you best. If you had been doing intermittent fasting for a long time, your body would automatically want to go back to its fasting stage once you divert away from it.

So look away from cheat days as you won't ever need them since you can consume whatever you want whenever you like it is as simple as that.

The Scale

When people decide to change their diet plans or health-related lifestyle, the first question they always end up asking is "how much weight can I lose?". Well, this all depends on your and your body.

When it comes to intermittent fasting, you should know it is not the first recommended choice for extreme weight loss or fast weight loss. There are many different factors that will come into play when it comes to weight loss.

You may be of the few people who end up losing up to ten pounds within a week, though in intermittent fasting, this fast of a result is rare but not impossible. You may even gain weight in the first week or two and think everything about intermittent fasting was a lie.

Realistically speaking, once your body has adjusted to this pattern of eating, you should be losing a pound per week. Start with a lower expectation and slowly build it up once you see results.

Remember, although what you eat won't matter as much during intermittent fasting, consuming more calories in than calories out will cause weight gain either way. The reason why there is a small feeding period kept in intermittent fasting is to reduce the number of calories you take in to balance out the number of calories you use.

But if you are capable of consuming more than a days' worth of calories even with a small eating period, then you may need to change some things within your diet.

However, do not keep the scale as your main way of knowing whether or not you are reaching your goal as you may just have gained weight due to a hearty meal or water retention from the pizza you ate last night.

Ideal Intermittent Fasting Plan

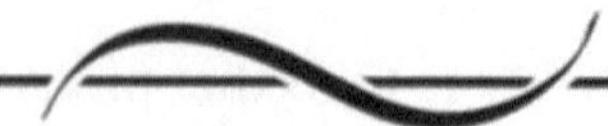

The ideal intermittent fasting plan depends entirely on you. There is no restriction behind what diet you should pick since every diet available in the intermittent fasting plan is different.

You are given so many choices for a reason; it is so that you can pick what works best for you. You can choose not to eat half the day and eat at night or the other way around as well.

Someone who is new to this type of diet should try a little of everything. Keep up a schedule for at least a month before you decide to drop it because it's said it takes you thirty days to build up a habit; some say fifteen but, let's stick to thirty for this one.

Get to know the different types of plans available for you just by reading the six plans made for you so you can get an idea of what you wish to do. Remember, if you think you are capable of creating your own plan, then do it! There is no harm in trying something that you are confident in.

Alternate day fasting (ADF)

Alternate day fasting has a 36-hour period of fasting and a 12 hour feeding time.

So, during an alternate day fasting, you fast almost every other day. This method of intermittent fasting has several other versions as well. Some of these versions involve consuming zero food for 24 hours, and for the rest of the 12 hours, you may consume a certain amount of calories.

Another version of this fast involves you only consuming up to five hundred calories on the days you have to "fast."

Many research studies used this method of intermittent fasting, sometimes alternating between different versions, and several of them showed health benefits.

As a beginner, it is best to stay away from this fast as it is not recommended for beginners or use its easier alternate versions.

This method of intermittent fasting requires a lot of self-control as with this method, you are going to be feeling extremely hungry several days per week.

Feeling hungry most days is not pleasant and can be very off-putting; this is why this method of fasting may be unsustainable in the long term.

To make this simple for you, all you have to do is start from Monday, eat for only 12 hours (let's take from 9 am to 9 pm) but do not try to binge as that is unhealthy. Then for the rest of Monday night as well as on Tuesday, you will not consume any food. After Tuesday, you can eat food on Wednesday, and the cycle continues.

On alternate day fasting, people are encouraged to make good food choices that are filling and healthy for the body. However, there is no restriction in this plan, so you can eat whatever you like when you are not fasting.

Here is a small schedule you can follow if you do not know how you must make your schedule:

Day 1	Day 2	Day 3	Day 4	Day 5	Day 6	Day 7
Eat for 12 hours	Fast for 24 hours Or Eat only a few calories during your "fast."	Eat for 12 hours	Fast for 24 hours Or Eat only a few calories during your "fast."	Eat for 12 hours	Fast for 24 hours Or Eat only a few calories during your "fast."	Eat for 12 hours

Meal-skipping

You do not always have to follow a strict schedule that will tell you when to eat and when to stop eating. For a successful intermittent fasting plan, you can receive all the benefits even though meal-skipping.

This may sound extreme to you as this behavior is associated with those who have eating disorders. However, meal skipping is not that hard to do; in fact, you may have been doing it without even knowing.

You do not need to skip meals every day; you can be skipping meals every other day. If you have dinner on Monday, skip breakfast on Tuesday, it's as simple as that. Keep these meal skips for days where you are too busy to cook or eat anything. This way, you won't suffer from any sort of malnutrition over the course of this fast since when you are busy, you tend to not consume any food either way.

You often hear this myth that tells you to consume food every few hours. This myth is not true unless you hit starvation mode or are losing muscle mass.

Remember, the human body is well equipped to handle fasts. Our body can go up to a maximum of two weeks to a month without proper food but even this length of time depends on the individual fat storage. So missing one or two meals a day is not a big deal.

Thus, if you do not feel like eating any food, you can just skip breakfast and eat a proper lunch or dinner. Same with if you are traveling and are having a tough time finding a place to eat, then try doing a short fast for the day.

This method of intermittent fasting is more spontaneous and less planned. Just be sure to eat proper food during your meal times to compensate for the meal you skipped.

Many people believe that meal skipping is a good thing as we should try to adapt to the things our ancestors did. They say as humans, we should exercise the same as we once used to, along with eating the proper amount of food every day.

You can follow the given schedule below if you do not know when you should skip your meals and when you should be consuming food:

Day 1	Day 2	Day 3	Day 4	Day 5	Day 6	Day 7
Breakfast	Skip	Breakfast	Breakfast	Breakfast	Breakfast	Skip
Skip	Lunch	Skip	Lunch	Lunch	Lunch	Lunch
Dinner	Dinner	Dinner	Dinner	Skip	Dinner	Dinner

Eat Stop Eat

Eat stop eat has a 24 hour fast once or twice a week and an open window for eating every other day of the week where you do not fast.

During eating stop eat fasting, you will fast for at least once a week. For this, you need to eat sensibly, meaning you need to take in a proper amount of protein, reduce processed foods, and so on.

The whole week is flexible for you, so this means you can choose which day of the week you wish to fast in.

You can fast starting from Monday's breakfast to Tuesdays Breakfast. All you will have to do is consume all the food you want during your breakfast time on Monday and stop eating for the rest of the day until Tuesday morning breakfast. You can also do this for lunch and dinner.

When you take on this fast, it can be fairly easy compared to others as it can be done during the weekend when you do not even have to go to work.

If you want to know how this method of intermittent fasting got so popular, then you can look into a man named "Brad Pilon."

For him, this plan worked perfectly since he knew how to handle this fasting method in his daily schedule. The same way, once you master this method of fasting, you will know what and how you have to do things in order for you to properly in cooperate this diet into your daily life.

You are allowed to consume a few drinks during your fast, but you cannot eat solid food during your fasting period. Below is a list for which drinks you can have during your fast:

- Tea
- Coffee
- Zero-calorie beverages
- Water

Remember, there is no such restriction in this plan that stops people from taking medication.

If you are trying to lose weight, then it is very important for you to eat the same amount of food you would usually eat during your non-fasting days. You will want to shove all the world's food in your mouth after you had nothing for a whole day, but your body has a limit, and you should not cross it. Eat slowly even when you feel like you need to take big bites.

The only downside of this fasting method is that not consuming anything for 24 hours is tough for many individuals. You may have events or parties to attend during some weekdays, and you might not want to be the oddball that does not participate in anything.

But its fine all you have to do is start slowly. Even starting with a fast of fourteen to sixteen hours is good. You can up the number of hours every week or so.

Here is a table you can follow if you do not know which days of the week you should fast:

Day 1	Day 2	Day 3	Day 4	Day 5	Day 6	Day 7
Eat as you would on a normal day	Fast	Eat as you would on a normal day	Eat as you would on a normal day	Eat as you would on a normal day	Fast	Eat as you would on a normal day

Lean gains (16/8 method)

The lean gains protocol involves a 16-hour period of fasting and gives you up to 8 hours to consume any food you want.

An individual should fast for up to a minimum of fourteen hours and must restrict their eating time to at least a minimum of eight hours or a maximum of ten hours.

The eating window is not small as compared to many other forms of intermittent fasting since you can easily fit in two to three meals within a day. You may very well be consuming a proper amount of calories and nutrients within this time frame daily.

The lean gains protocol is also known as the 16/8 method, and it was popularized by a fitness expert named "Martin Berkhan."

This method of fasting is super simple as all you have to do is not eat anything during dinner and skip Breakfast. This obviously depends on the timings of your meals as the time frame of the fast can be longer if you eat dinner early and Breakfast late.

But let's take an example, let's say you eat your last meal at 8 pm and end up not eating till noon the next day. Without even knowing you are fasting for up to sixteen hours.

For women, the recommended time for fasting is fourteen to fifteen hours, as the majority do better with this set time frame. Men can extend it to sixteen hours, though even if a woman wishes to keep a fast up to sixteen hours, then she can.

If you are a grumpy person early in the morning and absolutely must have breakfast every day, then this may be a tough protocol for you to follow at the start. However, those who skip breakfast usually have this pattern of eating either way, so it won't be as hard for them.

You can consume liquid during this diet as well. The liquid you are allowed include:

- Water
- Tea
- Coffee
- Zero-calorie beverages

If you struggle with your fast, then consuming liquids might ease the process as it can help reduce your hunger. The majority of times, we confuse dehydration for starvation so remember that when you step into this protocol.

This method of intermittent fasting won't work if you end up eating junk the whole eight hours. Eating too much won't do you any good for any type of fast, so try and keep an eye on that.

The lean gains protocol uses fast along with workouts to help you burn fat. Martin Berkhan kept a proper protocol if you fast while you workout, it means:

- An increase in blood flow to fat cells
- An increase in epinephrine and norepinephrine
- A slight increase in metabolic rate
- A decrease in insulin levels
- For energy, fatty acids will be released

Martin Berkhan says that the fasting period is the best time to be losing stored fat as your body tends to burn body fat when it does not have proper calories from the daily food intake.

However, if you extend the timing of your fast further, then it can have an opposite effect on your health and fitness progress.

This is why Martin Berkhan suggested that an individual must consume as many growths and recovery nutrients as possible after the fast is over. Of course, this does not mean you should overeat as that can cause stomach problems.

After you are done exercising, your body becomes more active in terms of nutrient uptake and subsequent protein synthesis. Thus Berkhan recommends that you eat as much as you can after you are done fasting. So in shorts terms, eat your largest meal of the day right after you have finished exercising.

If you do not know what schedule you should follow for the lean gains protocol, then you can start with the given schedule below before you can come up with one that suits you:

	Day 1	Day 2	Day 3	Day 4	Day 5	Day 6	Day 7
Midnight 4 am 8 am	Fast	Fast	Fast	Fast	Fast	Fast	Fast
12 am	Meal one	Meal one	Meal one	Meal one	Meal one	Meal one	Meal one
4 pm	Meal two and last meal before 8 pm	Meal two and last meal before 8 pm	Meal two and last meal before 8 pm	Meal two and last meal before 8 pm	Meal two and last meal before 8 pm	Meal two and last meal before 8 pm	Meal two and last meal before 8 pm
8 pm Midnight	Fast	Fast	Fast	Fast	Fast	Fast	Fast

Warrior Diet

In this diet, you will have to fast for 20 hours, and you will only be given 4 hours to eat food.

For the warrior diet, you either fast or eat only small portions of specific foods that have been recommended; this has to be done for the first 18 to 20 hours of the day, and you must work out during this period of fasting to see proper results.

Then for 4 to 6 hours, you will get to eat the majority of your daily food intake. Then again, for the next 18 to 20 hours, you will be fasting (and eating really small portions of food).

Most people like to keep their overfeeding period at the end of the day since it is more feasible for them to go into social settings such as family dinners, parties, and drinking with colleagues. But you can make any modifications you want. If you want, you can keep your 4 hour eating period during lunchtime or even Breakfast.

This "diet" was made popular by the fitness expert named "Ori Hofmekler."

In terms of what you can consume during your fasting period, it should stay under the categories of raw fruits and raw vegetables. Then for your 4 hour feeding time, you can eat whatever you like.

The warrior diet is considered to be one of the most popular intermittent fasts, and many people vouch for it. If you do not know what schedule to follow when you first start this form of intermittent fasting, then you can follow the given schedule below:

	Day 1	**Day 2**	**Day 3**	**Day 4**	**Day 5**	**Day 6**	**Day 7**
Midnight 4 am 8 am 12 am	Eating a small portion of fruits and vegetable	Eating a small portion of fruits and vegetable	Eating a small portion of fruits and vegetable	Eating a small portion of fruits and vegetable	Eating a small portion of fruits and vegetable	Eating a small portion of fruits and vegetable	Eating a small portion of fruits and vegetable
4 pm 8 pm Midnight	Eat anything	Eat anything	Eat anything	Eat anything	Eat anything	Eat anything	Eat anything

5:2 diet

The 5:2 diet is fairly simple. You eat as you would normally for five days a week, and for the rest of the two days, you need to restrict your calories to 500-600.

The diet is also commonly known as the "Fast Diet." It was popularized by a man named Michael Mosley, who is a British journalist.

On average, women need to eat 1200 calories a day, while men need to eat 1300 calories per day. In the same way, during the 5:2 diets fasting days' women should consume 500 calories and men need to consume 600.

However, if a woman has high muscle mass, then it is recommended that she too consume up to 600 calories during their fast.

You can choose any two days of the week where you wish to fast. There can even be a gap between the two days. So if you fasted on Monday, then you can keep the next fast on Friday.

There are not many studies available of 5:2 diet, but since it is a part of intermittent fasting, it is still capable of providing the same benefits.

If you do not know what schedule to make or follow for the 5:2 diet, then you can follow the given schedule below:

Day 1	Day 2	Day 3	Day 4	Day 5	Day 6	Day 7
Eat as usual	Consume only 500 (for women) to 600 (for men) calories	Eat as usual	Eat as usual	Eat as usual	Consume only 500 (for women) to 600 (for men) calories	Eat as usual

Weight Loss Through Intermittent Fasting

The basics behind intermittent fasting are that it allows the body to burn the stored energy in the body. This stored energy is kept in the form of fats, and when you go through a caloric deficit, then your body starts to use up the fats to make up for this deficit.

Body fat is simply energy that has been stored in your body for later use. If you stop eating, then your body will basically start "eating" itself to make up for the lack of energy.

The basic concept of fat is important and must be understood as it is part of the human body, and it is a natural thing. Humans have evolved and are capable of going through a long period of time without consuming any food.

You can see life has a way of making itself balance out things, both the good and the bad. The same idea is the basis of fasting since fasting has its bad sides (hunger), but it also has its good sides (the several health benefits).

So, here are how things work in our body:

When you eat food, you receive energy. You pretty much ingest energy. If the energy you have consumed is a little over the amount your body needed, it will store it for later use. Remember, the stored energy is really important, so do not think your body fat percentage should be extremely low.

Behind all of this, insulin is the key. Insulin is a hormone that is used for storing food energy within your body. Here's a small "diagram" to make things easy for you:

Consume food ▶ Increase in insulin ▶ storage of sugar and production of fat in the liver

Insulin production rises once we start to eat; this is so that it can help the body store the excess energy in two ways. The carbohydrates you consume are broken down into glucose, which is later stored in the liver or your muscles.

However, the liver and muscles have very little storage space to keep all those carbohydrates, so the body turns them into fat. This process has a unique name: De-novo lipogenesis. De-novo lipogenesis literally means making new fat.

Out of all that new fat that your body made, only some is stored in the liver. But the majority of it is kept as a fat deposit within your body, and this fat deposit is what makes our body grow larger. Our body can store a large amount of fat, and it can keep going until the body dies due to obesity-related health issues

So you can see the body has two storage systems. One is a more accessible option but has very little space. The other has a lot of space but is not as easily accessible. Below is a small diagram to show you the effect of fasting and what the simplest way to teach this process looks like:

Fasting (not eating food) ▶ Decrease in insulin ▶ body burns stored fat and sugar

As you can see above, the process can easily be reversed once you start to fast. When your blood sugar falls, your body will pull glucose out from stored energy. Thus, your body will start using its stored fat, and insulin level will drop if you are in fasting mode.

The glycogen in your body is the easiest energy source to access, and we get this source once carbohydrates are broken down into glucose and form a chain known as glycogen. While in energy storage, a chain is made in energy usage, the chain is broken back again to its original form, which is glucose.

Your stored glycogen has enough energy to give your body for 24-36 hours if you do not consume food. After this source is used up, the body will start to break down fats.

So as you can see, naturally, the body exists in two states, one is the fed state, and the other is the fasted state. We either increase our energy storage or decrease it. Now decreasing it may sound like it's a bad thing, but an excess amount of energy is a waste for the body as it can only use so much of it.

To restore your body's balance or to lose weight, all you have to do is increase the number of calories used per day. This can easily be done through intermittent fasting.

Since your body is not going to be in the fed state, and it will be in the fasted state, it will use up stored energy. Even animals have a long period of fasting known as hibernating. This is why they gain weight and then lose it during their hibernation period.

Eating every third hour is the recommended amount. Now, this does not mean eating full meals every three hours. It is more of a small snack with your proper meals. If you lack this balance in eating patterns, then intermittent fasting is meant for you.

Benefits of Intermittent Fasting

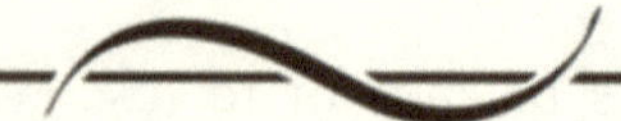

Of course, no one would recommend something to you if it did not have benefits. The same goes for intermittent fasting. You did not read all this way to find out that, in reality, it does not have much use. But don't worry because intermittent fasting has several benefits that can change your life for the better.

To know about them in more detail, read through the following benefits so that you can know why intermittent fasting has become such a hype.

Lowers Risk of Type 2 Diabetes

Type 2 diabetes is not something you haven't heard at this point in life as it has become increasingly common in many countries.

Type 2 diabetes involves a patient having high blood sugar levels as insulin resistance is increased. Any method that can reduce insulin resistance and helps lower a patient's blood sugar levels is great when it comes to type 2 diabetes.

Now when it comes to intermittent fasting, it does exactly what needs to be done for type 2 diabetes patients. Intermittent fasting has a huge effect on reducing insulin resistance and has shown to improve people's blood sugar levels.

Reduces Oxidative Stress and Inflammation

Oxidative stress hormones cause a lot of chronic diseases and bring you a step closer to aging. What is done by oxidative stress hormone is that it damages important protein and DNA molecules in your body.

Many studies have shown that oxidative stress hormones are reduced by intermittent fasting. Research has also shown that inflammation is also reduced due to intermittent fasting.

Lower Risk of Heart Disease

Heart diseases are the world's most common reasons for death.

Intermittent fasting is said to reduce the risk factor of several heart diseases by stabilizing blood pressure, improving LDL cholesterol, and improving blood sugar levels.

Cellular Repair

When you start to fast, your body will go into a cellular waste removal process; this process is known as autophagy. Autophagy involves breaking down the cells, metabolizing broken proteins, as well as dysfunctional proteins.

An increase in the levels of autophagy provides protection against several diseases. These diseases include cancer as well as Alzheimer's disease.

Prevent Cancer

Cancer is one of the toughest diseases to fight against. It is caused due to the uncontrollable growth of cells. Intermittent fasting has shown to have several effects on metabolism, and this can help reduce the risk of cancer.

There are many promising studies that have been held to prove that intermittent fasting can help reduce the cause of cancer. There are studies that have shown that fasting during chemotherapy has reduced various side effects related to it.

Brain Health

The majority of the time, whatever suits the body will suit the brain as well. Intermittent fasting has been proven to improve the body's metabolic features. An improvement in the body's metabolic rate also causes an improvement in the brain as well.

This improvement includes a reduction in the oxidative stress hormone, reduction in inflammation, and a reduction in insulin resistance.

Intermittent fasting is also said to increase the growth of nerve cells, which is beneficial for the brain as it will increase brain function.

Intermittent fasting also increases a brain hormone known as a brain-derived neurotrophic factor. A reduction in brain-derived neurotrophic hormone is said to have side effects such as depression and other brain problems.

Prevent Alzheimer's Disease

The world's most common neurodegenerative disease is known as Alzheimer's disease. Up till now, still has been no cure for Alzheimer's disease, so instead of looking for a cure after you've already gotten it, try taking measures to prevent it.

There have been several pieces of research and studies held to prove that intermittent fasting does have a positive effect on an individual's health, and this also includes positive effects for Alzheimer's disease.

In a study, those who fasted showed an improvement in their symptoms for Alzheimer's disease.

In some animal studies, it was suggested that protection against neurodegenerative diseases such as Parkinson's and Huntington's disease is increased for those who practice fasting. However, more studies need to be held for humans

Extend Lifespan

Everyone wants to live longer. Every diet plan suggests that once you follow it, you will extend your living years by ten more years. Many people dream of living above the age of 100 and still being able to move around peacefully.

Well, guess what? Intermittent fasting does just that. It is known to extend one's lifespan due to healthier eating choices and a better lifestyle.

A study on rats had shown that intermittent fasting could help extend people's lives. This is due to the continuous calorie restrictions that help us stay on track with healthy, filling foods.

In some other rat studies, the result of intermittent fasting was very shocking as one of the rats that had fasted every other day ended up living eighty-three percent longer than other rats who did not fast.

Although this does not prove anything in humans, it is still a great discovery as things that match with rats also match with humans. This is why intermittent fasting has become increasingly popular among people interested in anti-aging related products and practices.

Tips for Beginners

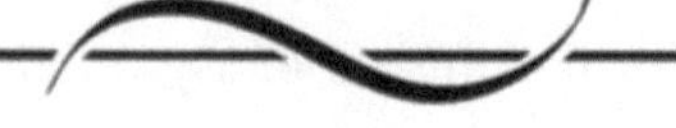

Maybe this is your first time entering intermittent fasting. Maybe it isn't, or your first time did not go as well, so you decided, "let's give it another chance," but this time with a guide. Either way, you are going to be a beginner, and everything can be a bit difficult for beginners.

You will receive several tips from people around you. Hopefully, those motivated you to work harder to reach your goal. The tips for intermittent fasting are basic but should be applied in your daily life to the best of your abilities so that you do not end up giving up on it.

So here are some tips to follow for you to become an expert in intermittent fasting:

Try Fasting After Dinner

One of the best tips anyone can give you is to start fasting after dinner. This has got to be one of the greatest tips you can follow in order to make things easier for yourself.

Make up any schedule that you like but always make sure that fasting after dinner is a part of it.

If you pick up this strategy, you spend the majority of your time sleeping through the hunger rather than being awake to suffer through all the self-control.

For example, let's say you are following the lean gains protocol. In it, you spend eight hours sleeping, which is the recommended amount of time one should be sleeping. You have already finished half your fast by sleeping through it, and now you will only need to go through eight more hours.

This method is really efficient since it makes you feel like you have cut down your work by half.

Plus, if you look at the lean gains protocol, you will be having your last meal at 8 pm, and then you will be going to sleep by 12 pm. These are the ideal timings, so when you look at it this way, you won't get hungry from 8 pm to 12 am since it is just a 4 hours' gap.

So at the end of the day, you would only really be going through 4 hours of "hunger" while the rest is something you won't even have to worry about. If you do feel like you would get hungry, then this is great practice for you since this is exactly something you are trying to fix.

Physiologically speaking, this will make you feel like your fast went by really fast and very easily. So, the easier it is for you to handle your fast, the easier it will be to continue on with this plan.

Difference between Boredom and Hunger

Before you start fasting, you need to know the difference between boredom and hunger.

Oftentimes, people end up consuming a lot of food just because of boredom; you might go grab a bar of chocolate here, a packet of chips, maybe even a glass of ice-cold soda. But this is something people do because people confuse boredom with hunger.

Through intermittent fasting, you are forcing yourself to stop equating boredom with hunger. You will only have the option to consume food during a certain period of time, and once you are past that timing, you will have to stop eating.

Through this, you will come to realize how much food you ate just because you were bored and had nothing to do.

Drink Water

For several people, when they go on to follow any diet or diet plan, the first thing they have in mind is losing weight.

Instantly when they think of weight loss as their only goal, they think that they must not include food or drinks at all.

However, this isn't a healthy thing to do, especially if you and fasting. This is because intermittent fasting isn't a short-term diet where once you lose 5 pounds, you stop doing it all together. No, intermittent fasting is a lifestyle and needs to be in cooperated into your daily life.

This is why you need to make sure that you are drinking enough water when you are fasting. Keeping a higher water intake will allow you to also suppress your appetite.

So not only are you being healthy by not continuously shoving food in your mouth, but you are also helping yourself stay hydrated.

If you're wondering how much water you should consume in a day, then just follow these simple steps:

- Measure your weight
- Divide it by 2
- The answer you get is the amount of water you should be drinking in one day

Skip Flavored Drinks

While it is important to stay hydrated when you are fasting, it does not mean you should be drinking everything you lay your eyes on.

Hydration is only meant to be done through water or electrolyte drinks (when participating in sports). Stay away from sugary drinks such as flavored juices, powdered juice mixes, and sodas. Even if the product says it is sugar-free or low in sugar, still do not consume it.

All of these flavored drinks are filled with artificial sweeteners that aren't just bad for your health, but they make you feel even hungrier over time.

The majority of these drinks will make you feel even hungrier. Thus it is better to keep up your diet after you have come so far along, rather than ruining it over something as cheap are flavored drinks.

Consume Protein

When you are fasting, one of the hardest things to maintain is your protein intake. This is due to several reasons, such as:

- First, proteins tend to be satiating. This means you get full more easily.
- Secondly, because you have a limited time to eat your food, you do not get enough time to eat the necessary proteins.

But, during intermittent fasting, you need to make sure that you are taking in enough protein to maintain your muscle mass. There is no use of fasting if you are losing weight in the form of muscles; your aim should be to reducing body fat, not body muscle mass.

Losing muscle mass will make you feel weaker, and your resting metabolic rate will start to decrease, meaning the number of calories you burn just doing minimum movements will become much lesser than before.

This is why protein intake is so important. Generally speaking, your aim should be consuming up to 30% protein daily. Do not just take your protein in powder form; look into a protein-filled vegetable, chicken, and seafood.

Avoid Unhealthy Foods

One of the biggest mistakes people make during intermittent fasting is just focusing on eating food and not focusing on what kind of food they should be eating.

Fasting for more than eight hours a day does not give you an excuse to eat almost anything and everything. So do not just consume junk foods when you are finished with fasting.

You can eat junk food if you want. It's not like you need to cut it out fully out of your diet. But eating junk food, the majority of the time, will be hard as you must take proper nutrients within a small time frame.

It is difficult to stop right away, but you do not need to give up instantly. However, you will have to make some sort of effort to perfect this lifestyle.

Make this change slowly, and you will succeed at it. Do it instantly, and you will have issues with it.

Take it Slow

One of the biggest mistakes people make is starting to fast all the way without stepping into it slowly.

In many cases, people end up going back to their old way because having such a change is hard, and they want to go back to things that were easier for them since they had been practicing it for years.

But this is not the long term solution. Intermittent fasting is not a diet, but it is a lifestyle. The best approach to take is easing yourself into this plan.

It can take people months to get used to intermittent fasting. But once you have succeeded at it, you won't ever want to go back as this is the simplest way to keep your health in check.

Let's take the lean gains protocol as an example; when you start your first day, instead of skipping Breakfast, delay the timing at which you normally eat your Breakfast.

You can keep the delay time as thirty minutes and gradually take this time up every day until your Breakfast turns into your lunchtime.

These small tricks will help you get used to fasting quickly without making you have a mental breakdown or making you want to shift back to your old ways.

Who Shouldn't Try Intermittent Fasting?

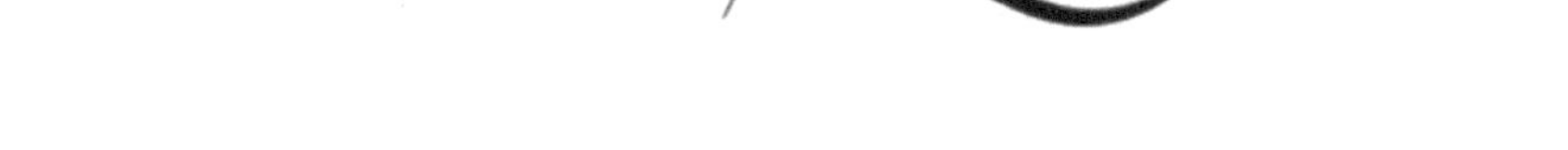

Out of every diet plan, you would have tired; intermittent fasting is going to be the easiest to follow. Several people love it because of this very reason. It is not complicated and has so many versions that can suit almost every person in the world.

This is the least mentally draining way of reaching your lifestyle goals, and several studies have also shown the amazing effect intermittent fasting has had on people's lives. You, too, must have read about them.

However, intermittent fasting is not made for everyone; in fact, there are several people that should avoid intermittent fasting. The following is a list of people who should not try intermittent fasting, along with why they should not try it:

People Suffering from an Eating Disorder

Intermittent fasting requires people to follow a strict plan and needs people to eat only in a small time frame. This can be extremely triggering for those suffering from eating disorders such as bulimia or binge eating disorder. Before you to start intermittent fasting, check in with a doctor to evaluate your mental health first.

Pregnant Women

Pregnancy is hectic and can take a big toll on a woman's body. Many say pregnancy means eating for two, but of course, in moderation. Nevertheless, the number of calories you consume may go up by a percentage, but they will never go down since women are carrying another tiny human in them.

Fasting can lead to low blood sugar and energy level. It can also cause a lack of nutrition for the baby. During pregnancy, you need to be getting good nutrition and proper food intake, not anything else.

People suffering from Type 1 Diabetes

Although intermittent fasting is amazing for type 2 diabetes patients, it is not the best thing for those suffering from type 1 diabetes. Type 1 diabetes patients are dependent on insulin, and having to adapt to one diet plan can be difficult.

If someone with type 1 diabetes does not consume food for a day or even for half a day, their blood sugar can go down to dangerous levels. This is why intermittent fasting is not recommended for type 1 diabetes patients.

Athletes in Training

Although doing an everyday workout while fasting is okay, it becomes not okay when you are a training athlete, as you will be using up a lot of calories in one day. If your calorie intake per day is less than the calories you use, it can reduce your performance in sports. Sports that require a lot of cardio also require proper food intake, so if you are someone who is training, then it is best not to start intermittent fasting.

Side Effects of Intermittent Fasting

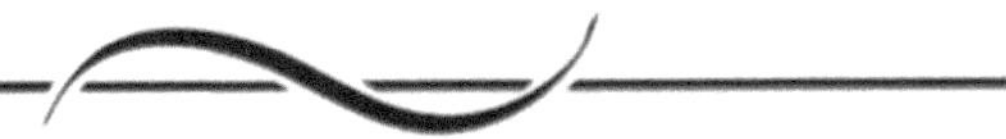

Although intermittent fasting has a lot of benefits, it also has a lot of side effects. As with any change in lifestyle, intermittent fasting can also have a few negative effects. So here are a few of them along with their solution:

1. Hunger

Hunger is one of the biggest side effects of intermittent fasting. This won't be an issue you will face if you already were trying diets that were low in the carb or higher in fat.

2. Constipation

If you eat less, it means you will remove less. But this is normal since you are not eating a lot of food. It is not a huge concern, so you do not need to seek treatment for it unless you are getting bloated or have abdominal discomfort.

You can use standard laxatives or even magnesium supplements to reduce the discomfort if needed.

3. Headaches

Headaches are normal as well and will disappear once you get used to the fasting schedule. You can take some salt to help with the headaches.

Overall you should drink mineral water to help with your stomach issues. Other side effects can include dizziness, heartburn, and muscle fatigue.

 The most serious side effect you might face is a refeeding syndrome. This is really rare and only happens if you fast for 5 to 10 days or more. The chances of refeeding syndrome increases if someone is undernourished and is also fasting.

The majority of these side effects have easy solutions, so this should not stop you from keeping your fasts. However, if you feel unwell and do not think you can continue your fast, then, of course, you are allowed to break it.

Just remember to eat slowly once you have broken your fast and first try to take a bite of more fluid foods rather than the solid food. But don't worry too much because severe side effects are rare.

Frequently Asked Questions

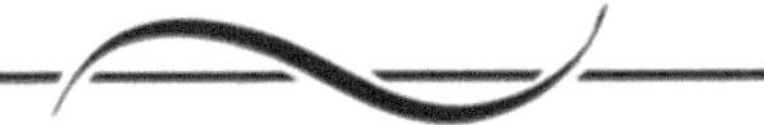

Can I Drink Liquids While Fasting?

Yes, you are allowed to drink liquids while you fast. However, you need to limit the liquids to tea, coffee, water, and non-caloric beverages. You cannot add any sugar to these drinks, but you can add a small amount of milk or cream.

Is it Unhealthy to Skip Breakfast?

No, it is not unhealthy to skip breakfast. The only issue related to breakfast skippers is that majority of them do not have a healthy lifestyle. If you make sure not to binge and eat the proper amount of food per day, it should not matter.

Can I Take Supplements While Fasting?

You are allowed to take supplements. However, fat-soluble vitamins are said to work better when taken with a meal.

Can I Exercise While Fasting?

There are no restrictions for training while you fast as the majority versions of intermittent fasting allow for water and liquid intake. However, some people recommend taking branched-chain amino acids (BCAAs) before you start your workout while fasting

It is also recommended that if you perform aerobic exercises, you should eat a meal before the workout as it increases the performance. Also, take in fluids that and some sodium (salt) when you are fasting.

Will I Lose My Muscles If I Fast?

Almost every weight-loss method can cause muscle loss; this is why it is important for you to keep up your training and take in enough protein. There are different versions of intermittent fasting that can be followed in order to avoid muscle loss.

The amount of muscle loss a person faces is dependent on what they consume during their diet. An increase in protein intake should be the number one priority if you wish to gain muscle mass.

Will Fasting Slow Down My Metabolism

No, it will not. In fact, intermittent fasting increases an individual's metabolic rate.

Will I suffer from starvation mode?

Starvation is not a part of intermittent fasting; in fact, it is the biggest myth about it. Of course, this myth is not true as several pieces of research have shown that intermittent fasting can increase an individual's metabolic rate and is also capable of improving overall body health.

Can my child try intermittent fasting?

No, they are still growing and need proper nutrition every hour of the day. Thus, letting your child fast is not a good idea as even their metabolism levels are higher than adults.

Conclusion

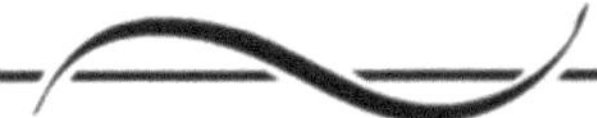

Any plan or any diet that you keep will work well if it is done for yourself and for your own health before anything else. You are likely to be demotivated if you start doing something because of what others have said.

This fact is important to understand when you step into the world of intermittent fasting. Weight loss should not be your only goal. Fixing any sort of health issue should be your first priority. Engaging in good physical activities along with a healthy diet is the best lifestyle you can ask for.

www.ingramcontent.com/pod-product-compliance
Lightning Source LLC
Chambersburg PA
CBHW051132250726
48655CB00007B/3012